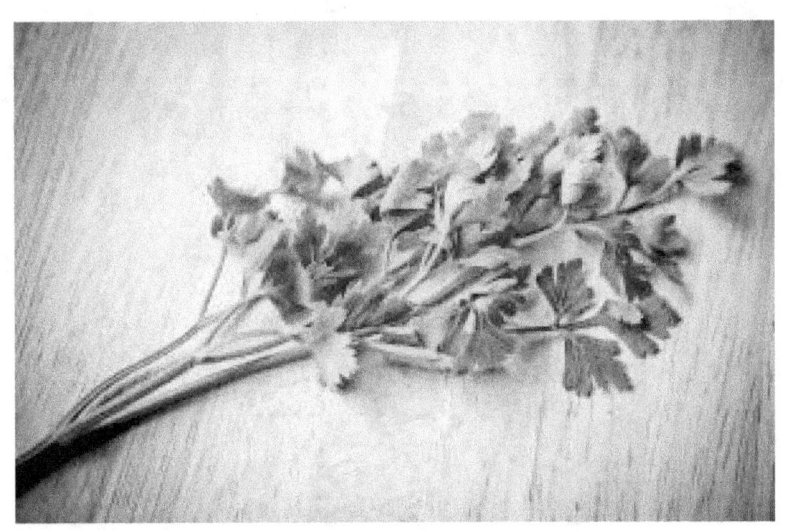

Chinese Medicinal Plants

How to Grow Them, How to Use Them

Published By Shaharm Publications

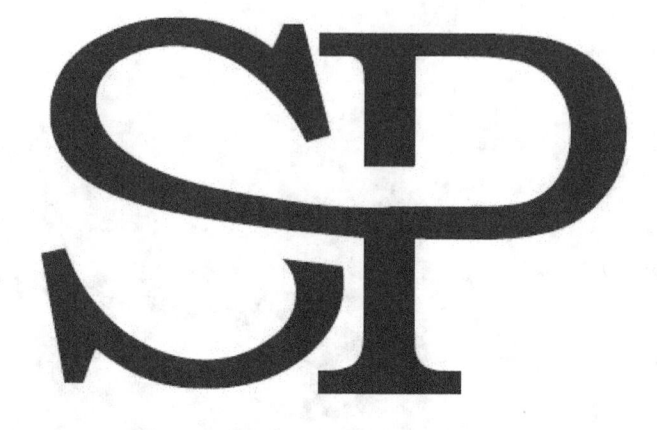

SHAHARM PUBLICATIONS

For a full list of books by Shaharm Publications, please go to:

http://www.shaharmpublications.com

Table of Contents

1. Is Healing with Plants Possible?

All of us are concerned about our health, regardless of whether we are experiencing a health difficulty at this time or if we just want to make sure that we enjoy life because of the level of health that we experience. In either case, there are options available to assist you in caring for your health properly. One of those options is to take advantage of some of the ancient Chinese medical knowledge that comes from plant-based healing. That is what this publication is designed to do, to help you to enjoy what the plants around us have to offer.

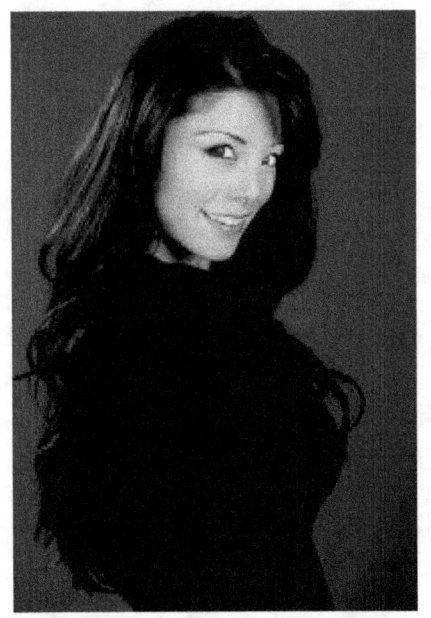

In this book, we will discuss many factors that will allow you to enjoy a higher level of health. From the different types of plants that can assist you in experiencing better health to understanding how to grow those plants effectively, it will all be explained to you so that you can begin this exciting and healthy hobby as well. Although many different factors will be considered, the following subjects are going to be discussed in greater detail for your benefit.

History - One important factor that we will consider in this publication is the history of ancient Chinese medication. Admittedly, with it being thousands of years old, much of the information has been lost to time, but understanding what is still available can help you to appreciate what this ancient form of healing has to offer. You will be amazed with what the culture was able to accomplish without the use of modern technology, something that often hampers us more than it helps us. Taking a look at the history of plant-based medication can heighten your appreciation for it.

Benefits - More than likely, you are looking for some specific types of benefits when it comes to the natural medication that is available through various plants. Perhaps you are looking to overcome some physical ailment, or it may be a mental or emotional difficulty that needs to be treated. Those are specific benefits, and they are going to be discussed in greater detail in Chapter 3. You will also find that there are additional benefits that you may not have considered possible. Looking into all of the benefits can provide you with the motivation necessary to get started.

Gardening - Although it is possible to buy many of the herbs and other plants that can be used for healing at local vitamin shops or online, it is not always the best option to do so. In some cases, you need to be concerned about the quality of the products that you are purchasing. In addition, you have to wonder if the potency of those products is going to be what is necessary to provide you with the healing that you need.

Because of the possibility of receiving low-quality or low potency products when you purchase them through a commercial resource, growing them yourself is an option that you will want to consider. We will look at some of the ways that you can grow a healing garden at home. You will be amazed with how easy it is to get started, and you can grow your own garden outdoors or you can even grow it indoors to enjoy what it has to offer every day of the year.

Top Plants - There are dozens, if not hundreds of different plants that can be grown for the healing properties that they offer. Although it would be nice to grow these plants individually, it is not always feasible to grow all of them. Perhaps you are limited by space or it may be a matter of being limited by time. That is why we will discuss the top medicinal plants and what they may be able to do for you and your health. Additionally, we will talk about how easy it is for you to grow some of these plants and you may wish to consider incorporating many of them into your own healing garden.

When You Can't Grow - Although it would be ideal if you could grow all of your own medicinal herbs at home, doing so is not always going to be possible. Because of various limitations, we may find it necessary to purchase some of these plants through an outside resource. In Chapter 6 of this publication, we will talk about some of the best options for ordering products and making sure that you are getting the highest quality and highest potency options available. In that way, you can feel comfortable that you are getting the most benefit from the supplements that you are using.

Lifestyle - When you use medicinal plants as a regular part of your life, you will find that you are improving your overall health. There are also other things that can be done that will help to improve your health as well. It is really up to you to determine how many of the factors that are discussed in this publication will be incorporated into your life. By incorporating them regularly, however, you will find that you are able to live a healthier lifestyle and to enjoy more of what life has to offer.

Options - Medicinal plants are the primary focal point of this publication. Entire volumes could be written about the healing properties that plants have to offer, but it may not be the only part of Chinese medicine that you want to consider. The fact of the matter is that there are different options that have been in practice for thousands of years that you can incorporate in your life as a part of a healthier lifestyle. We will discuss some additional ancient Chinese medical options that are popular today.

Making the choice to live a healthier lifestyle will benefit you in a number of ways. If you are dealing with a specific illness, using the right herbs may be able to help you to feel better and some people have seen amazing benefits by using the right medicinal plants. If you're not yet experiencing serious medical problems and would like to avoid them, living a healthier lifestyle through ancient Chinese medical practices may be an option that you want to consider. By incorporating them into your lifestyle, you will likely experience benefits that are beyond what you had hoped for.

2. The Roots and Advancements of Chinese Medicine

Throughout history, many cultures have had a great interest in making sure that the level of health of the population was as high as possible. Many of those cultures, however, fell short when it came to treating people in a way that actually helped them. For thousands of years, those cultures have used various medical practices that actually hurt individuals. In fact, it could even be seen as recently as the 19th century, when leeches were used for treating a wide variety of medical problems, in many cases, to the detriment of those who were using them.

One culture that stood out from among the others was the Chinese culture. For about 5000 years, the Chinese have been using a form of natural healing practices to help individuals that were suffering from a wide variety of ailments. In fact, from writings that are well over 2000 years old, it was seen that those practices were well established, and they were even helpful, with many of the benefits seen for the long-term. What is even more interesting is the fact that many of the ancient Chinese theories of medication are still being used down to this day.

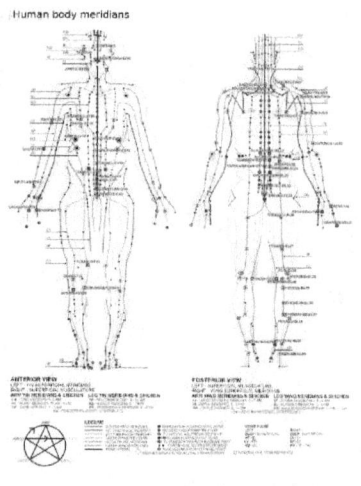

Throughout the world, a variety of Chinese medical practices are used in alternative forms of therapy. Some of these different types of therapies are going to be considered in another chapter of this publication and they include acupuncture and massage. The use of plant-based healing is also very common in Chinese culture, and it is something that is studied widely by people around the world today. In Western lands, the use of natural medicine, such as what is available through ancient Chinese medical practices is sometimes frowned on. In Eastern cultures, however, it is embraced by the medical community and it is often used right along with common medical practices of this day.

In order to understand more about Chinese medical practices and what they may be able to offer to your health, it is good to understand the basic principles of Chinese medicine. These principles may have changed from time to time throughout history but as far as we can tell, they are still very close to what was practiced thousands of years ago. Here are some of the basic principles that can help you to understand more about Chinese medication.

Methods of Diagnosis

There are 4 different methods of diagnosis that are used in Chinese medicine. Understanding these different methods of diagnosis can help you to get your start in understanding more about this medical culture as well. In many cases, using these methods of diagnosis will allow the physician that is caring for you to understand what is taking place and what needs to be done in order to treat it.

Observation - This is the first of the methods of diagnosis and it is rather straightforward. When you see a physician that understands the principles of Chinese medicine, he will first observe you from an exterior standpoint. Using various methods observation, he can recognize what is taking place on the inside by looking at what is taking place on the outside. In that way, anything that may be wrong internally, including problems with the internal organs or glands will show up in some way on the outside. It may be your skin color or perhaps some sign that shows in your eyes or on your face, but when the physician is skilled at recognizing the signs, he can learn a lot about your health through observation.

Sound and Smell - It is not only the outward appearance that allows the physician to know what is taking place inside the body, he will also use his sense of hearing and smell to determine if there is a problem. For example, the physician may listen to the sounds of you breathing, which can say a lot for any breathing difficulties that you may have. He may also listen for any sounds that are made by your digestive system. In some instances, the sense of smell is even more powerful, and it can help the doctor to know what is taking place. If you are experiencing a problem with an internal organ or gland, your body may produce a certain type of smell that will allow the doctor to know what is taking place internally.

Interrogation - With this step, the physician will go beyond the overall senses and what your body may be saying, and he will ask questions of you and perhaps even your relatives. This is typically done with a view to recognizing symptoms that you are experiencing and in seeing how the disease is evolving.

Palpation - The fourth method of diagnosis is done by taking the pulse on your radial artery. According to Chinese medical theory, if your body is healthy, the pulse is going to be steady and uninterrupted. If you are unhealthy, however, there will be variations in the quality of your pulse that can be detected by the physician.

The doctor will not rely on any single factor to determine what is taking place inside of the body. He will consider all four different methods of diagnosis and use a combination of the information that he has gathered to determine what is wrong and what can be done to treat any problems that exist.

Yin and Yang

Another basic principle of Chinese medicine is that of balance, sometimes referred to as Yin and Yang. According to the belief structure within ancient Chinese medicine, our bodies are constantly undergoing a give-and-take or a push and shove. There are negative forces within the body, known as the Yin and they are balanced by the positive external forces, known as Yang. As long as there is balance between Yin and Yang the body will be healthy. Anytime the body becomes unhealthy and disease is evident, it is thought to be due to a lack of harmony of these two relative properties.

Qi (Chi)

It is thought that there is a flow of energy in all living things. This energy flows throughout the living organism, and it produces life and sustains it. In ancient Chinese culture, this energy is known as Qi, or Chi. It is the life force within us and as long as it flows freely throughout the body, we are able to enjoy a balanced degree of health.

Chi is also thought to help to link things together, including all living organisms and even linking living organisms with their surroundings. It is the flow of energy that is often discussed in feng shui, and it is very important when it comes to ancient Chinese medical practices as well.

The human body has been mapped according to traditional Chinese medicine and there are certain patterns which show the flow of Qi along pathways within the body that are known as meridians. As long as this energy is flowing freely, the body is healthy. If there is any time when the energy is blocked or disrupted or if an imbalance occurs within the movement of the energy through the meridians, it can lead to illness.

If there is a disruption in the flow of Qi in the human body, there are a number of options available for freeing it according to traditional Chinese medicine. Some of those options include certain types of martial arts training, acupressure, and acupuncture and, as you will learn in this publication, herbology and food therapy.

The Advancement of Traditional Chinese Medicine

For thousands of years, traditional Chinese medicine has been used in the same form and with the same benefits without variation. Although there were times in ancient days in which things did change according to new knowledge that was understood, eventually, enough was known that could treat almost any ailment that was experienced. Therefore, traditional Chinese medicine has not advanced in the past several thousand years and it is still used in the same way as it was by those ancient physicians.

That isn't to say, however, that there are not any advancements that are beneficial in medicine. In Western cultures, those who are interested in using traditional Chinese medicine, including the use of food therapy and herbology, often scoff at Western medical science. In China, however, as well as in other Asian cultures, both are embraced and are used in conjunction with each other for all the benefits that they provide.

As is the case with anything in life, it is important to be balanced. Throwing all caution to the wind and simply trying to heal a serious illness with the use of herbs could be disastrous. On the other hand, ignoring what natural healing may have to offer to you could be disastrous as well. Being balanced in this regard, using what modern science and ancient practices have to offer is often the best course of action. Being balanced in this way will often yield the best results.

3. The Benefits of Using Plants for Healing

Modern science has really changed the way that many people look at medicine today. It wasn't all that long ago that a healing balm or an herb tea would have been recommended for almost any type of ailment, and in many cases it would have been accepted and seen great success. Today, however, many people forgo the possibility of using natural plants and methods of healing in favor of what science has to offer. Unfortunately, much of it also includes the use of prescription drugs and poisons, some of which are given unnecessarily and can cause severe health problems and side effects.

This publication is not designed to tell you to stop using what modern science has to offer. The fact of the matter is that there are many cases

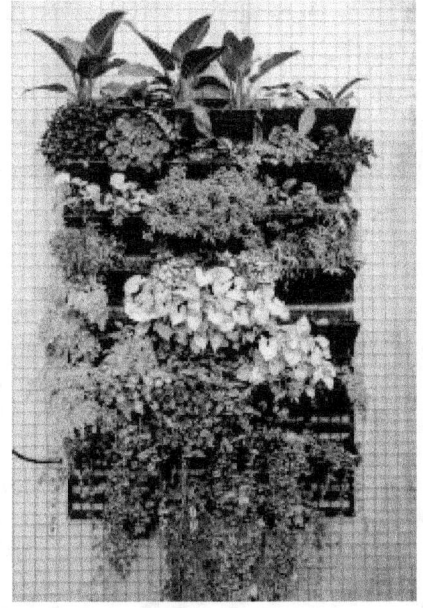

in which modern medical science can assist you in overcoming the problem and in dealing with it successfully. What you may want to consider doing, however, is being balanced in your view of medicine. At times, it may be possible to heal yourself through the use of herbs and other natural treatments, or at the very least you can use it to supplement the medical treatments that you are receiving. As long as the two don't contradict each other, using the best of both may be the best option that is available.

More than likely, you are already looking for a very specific benefit when it comes to using food therapy or some type of traditional Chinese medicine. For most people, it is an attempt to heal something specific that may be going on with their physical, mental or emotional health. Other individuals are simply trying to live a healthier lifestyle and they recognize that the use of herbal medication may be able to help in that regard. Although those benefits certainly do exist, there are other benefits to using plants for healing as well. We will discuss some of those benefits further in this chapter.

History - One of the benefits of using herbs for medicine is the fact that you are using something that has a long and celebrated history. In this publication, we are primarily focused on traditional Chinese medicine and the fact that they have been using food therapy and herbs for thousands of years. In reality, there have been many cultures that have used food as a form of healing and with great success. Included among those cultures are the Native American, Greek, and Egyptian cultures. All of them recognized the benefits of using herbs for healing, and those benefits still carry through till today.

Price - Unfortunately, many of us have a difficulty affording the medication and modern healthcare that we may need for our situation. In fact, many people have stopped using prescription drugs because they could not afford them. Although that may be necessary in some cases, you should always try to care for yourself in the best way possible. If all you can do is use an herbal remedy to treat the situation, it is something that should not be overlooked. Growing your own herbs and healing foods can provide you with those benefits on a budget.

Side effects - Most prescription medications and many modern medical treatments will have side effects that are associated with them. In some cases, the side effect may even be worse than the issue that is being treated in the first place. For example, many depression medications carry a side effect of possibly creating additional depression and suicidal thoughts. Those side effects do not exist when you use herbal medications. Of course, there may be some side effect from time to time but they are few and far between in comparison with what is seen through most prescription drugs.

Environment - Most of us have become environmentally aware and we want to ensure that we are caring for the environment in the best way possible. One way that we can do so is through the use of herbs and healing foods. As an example, when you take prescription medication for a health problem, some of the medication is going to end up in the sewage system and will even be recycled and be back into the water system again. It is estimated that there are hundreds of different chemicals forming a toxic soup in the drinking water in most areas. You do not have such a problem with herbs.

Options - Modern medical science and many of the drugs that are being prescribed are for a very specific use. In fact, there may even be multiple drugs that are prescribed for the same purpose, and your doctor will have to choose the one that is specific to your needs. When you use herbal medication, however, you tend to have more options because the herbs can be used for a variety of purposes. In some cases, you may choose to use food therapy for one reason and you will end up benefiting in many different ways as a result of using it.

Of course, these are just a few of the many different reasons why individuals use traditional Chinese medicine and herbal therapy. You will find that there are many other benefits that come your way, and they will become more evident as you begin to use the food for the medicinal benefits that it provides.

4. Planning Your Healing Garden

Obtaining herbs and other plants for their medicinal properties can be of benefit, but it is much more beneficial if you are able to grow them at home. After all, you have greater control over the quality of the medicinal plants that you are using if you are growing them. In addition, you will find that it is possible to save a considerable amount of money because medicinal plants can be expensive if they are purchased commercially. In this chapter, we are going to look at a few of the options available for growing medicinal plants at home and how you can get started in this exciting hobby.

First of all, it's important to recognize that many of the plants that you are growing were actually grown in the wild and were found outside of the cultivated land when they were first used. In some instances, you may still be able to find medicinal plants in the wild, but you need to be cautious and understand what you are doing before you start collecting them. There may be plants that are closely related to each other, with one being helpful and the other being poisonous. As a general rule, you should never use a wild plant unless you are absolutely sure you are using the right one.

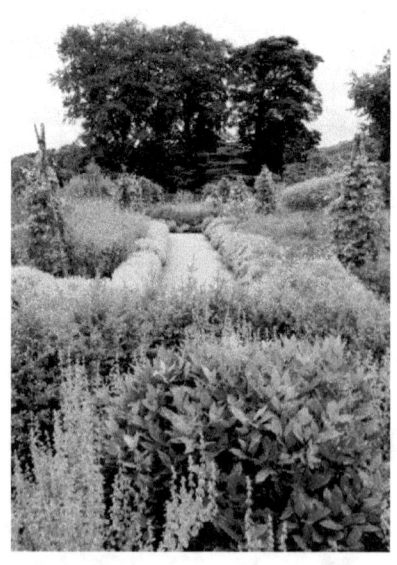

It is also important to recognize that not all medicinal plants are going to be able to be grown in all areas. In some cases, your climate is not going to support the growth of the plant, although you may still be able to grow it indoors, at least in a limited capacity. It is best if you try to grow the ones that are right for you and to put a greater emphasis on the plants that you will personally use. You may also want to branch out into some additional plants, if you have the time to do so.

If you are new to growing a garden and would like to get started successfully, it is best if you start simply. Although it will always be possible for you to expand on your garden a later time, it is best if you only grow the plants that you need at first until you see how you will do with the process. There are many different plants that can be grown successfully at home, but those that are the easiest to grow and the most beneficial include Echinacea, chamomile and peppermint. These plants will provide you with some of the basic health needs for your family and are relatively easy to grow.

Planning Your Garden

A number of things need to be considered when planning your garden to ensure that it has the greatest chance for success. You want to plant it in the right area of the property so that it has adequate sunlight but not too much sunlight for those plants that prefer partial shade. In addition, you want to ensure that you have easy access to the garden. It is much easier to tend the garden if it is nearby. Although it may be tempting to plant it in the far reaches of your property, if you have a rather large area available, it can make it difficult to work on it regularly.

A raised bed garden is the best choice if you are going to be growing your medicinal garden outdoors. You can build a raised bed garden out of any material, but it is best if you choose something that is not treated chemically. For example, you can build a raised bed out of 4 x 4's or landscaping timbers but it is best if you don't use pressure-treated wood or railroad ties, because the chemicals that are included in the wood could leach into the soil. Raised bed gardens provide you with easy access to the plants that you are growing, and they are much more manageable than allowing the garden to spread over a larger area.

Some of the plants that you are growing can be grown in odd areas of the property and don't necessarily need to be included in the general garden. For example, peppermint is easily grown in almost any area around the home and it will take on a life of its own once you get started.

There are many medicinal plants that have these types of properties and you will find that having little pockets of those plants here and there around the property is all that is really needed. You can then concentrate on some of the additional plants that are specific to your garden.

Pay particular attention to the quality of the soil, which is a step that is often skipped by home gardeners. When you first turn the soil in the springtime, it is best if you have it tested at a local co-op to see if it needs any treatment to get it balanced properly. Be cautious about the suggestions that they give you when it comes to balancing the soil, because they are likely to suggest chemical measures. There are always going to be organic options that can be considered.

Unlike a vegetable garden, which may need to be tended on a daily basis, a healing herb garden will not need as much attention. At times, you may find that a week or longer passes by and the garden will do quite well on its own. That is due to the nature of the plants that are being grown, as they are easily grown in the wild in many cases. Because they are hardy and tend to grow well on their own, a little bit of attention is all that is typically necessary to keep them going strong.

Feeding Your Garden

It is also a good idea for you to feed your herb garden on a regular basis. This is done by producing organic compost, something that is very easy to do. In order for compost to grow, it needs basic elements of air, organic material and moisture. If you have a small pile of organic material in the corner of your yard and keep the moisture content at a consistent level, you would be surprised with how quickly you can produce healthy compost. It can then be spread on the garden area in the fall and you will have a healthier and livelier garden in the following year.

Getting rid of any weeds that grow in the garden is also important. It is a good idea for you to get familiar with the different types of weeds that grow in your area, as some of them may be beneficial for medicinal use as well. Some of the weeds may also be poisonous, so you need to know the difference before you use them. Tending to the weeds regularly will help your garden grow because it will get rid of the competition in the area and allow your healing herbs to thrive.

Growing Your Garden Year-Round

Although much of the focus for growing herb gardens is going to be outdoors, it is also possible to grow many of the herbs indoors. Growing an indoor garden is relatively easy and only takes a small corner of your room or perhaps a windowsill or two, and you will have plenty of herbs that can be used for healing balms and tea throughout the year.

As is the case with growing your garden outdoors, it is important to start small when it comes to growing an indoor garden as well. Many people prefer to start by growing a few plants on a windowsill in the kitchen. As long as you provide sunlight for the plants and keep the soil moist, you would be surprised with how easy it is to grow these plants indoors.

It is also possible to increase your efforts and to have an even greater indoor growing season. If you have the space available for it, you can purchase some grow lights and grow additional plants indoors 365 days a year. This is an excellent choice for those who have a specific health need and want to make sure that they have the highest quality plants available for medicinal purposes. Growing a few plants in the garage, in a closet or even in a corner of the room is possible and it will provide you with an ongoing supply of medicinal herbs.

Each plant that is grown is going to have its own, unique properties. Many of the plants that are grown for medicinal use are very easy to grow and some will even grow on their own quite heartily without any extra effort on your part. Other plants, however, tend to be rather delicate and are going to need additional work on your part in order to get them growing well. With a little bit of effort, however, it is possible to grow a beautiful garden indoors or outdoors and have the medicinal plants that you need for the needs of your family.

5. The Top Medicinal Plants and How to Grow Them

When it comes to traditional Chinese medicine and the use of herbs and plants for healing, you are not limited when it comes to options. In fact, it can sometimes be difficult to decide which of the options you are going to use. In this chapter, we are going to focus in on the top medicinal plants that are typically grown for their health benefits. You will likely find some of these will make an excellent addition in your own garden and others may be something that you want to experiment with at some time in the future.

Evening Primrose – Many parts of the evening Primrose plant can be used for healing benefits. The roots and shoots can be made into a poultice for the treatment of bruising and hemorrhoids. It is also possible to make a tea from the roots that will help to relieve digestive upset and 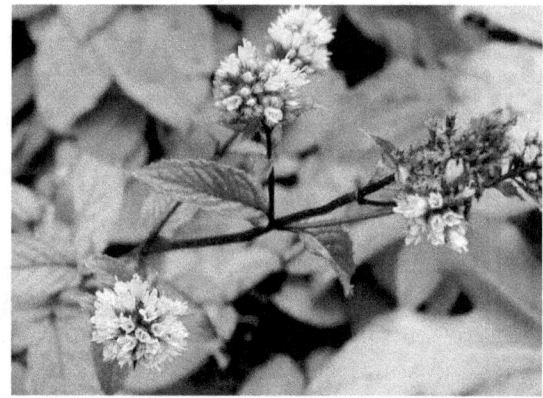 may help you to lose weight as well. In most cases, however, it is the bark and the leaves that are used for the production of Primrose oil. Primrose oil is used for treating a wide range of problems, including multiple sclerosis, eczema, hyperactivity, acne and arthritis. Although it is considered to be a weed, it can also be grown in a controlled environment, even indoors.

Goji Berry - This remarkable plant produces a berry that can be used in a wide variety of foods and has unique and helpful health properties. In some environments, it is possible to grow it outdoors, but it is better if you grow it in your indoor garden, perhaps even growing it on a windowsill. It is a perennial, so once you get it growing, it is likely to provide you with an ongoing harvest for quite some time.

Mushrooms - There are hundreds of species of mushrooms in traditional Chinese medicine that you may want to consider using. Unfortunately, some of these mushrooms can be difficult to grow in a regular garden. They are still worth mentioning, however, because of the possibilities that they have of treating a wide variety of issues that you may be facing.

Peppermint – This plant is perhaps one of the better known of the medicinal plants that is used in traditional Chinese medicine and throughout the world. It is very easy to grow and in the right climate, you can simply plant some in an out-of-the-way corner of the yard and harvest it as needed. The leaves have an aromatic property that provides benefits and when crushed and rubbed on the skin, can help to relax the muscles. It is also possible to make a tea from the leaves that will help to treat everything from fevers to an upset stomach and irritable bowel syndrome.

Tea Tree - More than likely, you have used tea tree oil at some time in the past. It has antibacterial and antifungal properties and is often used as an antiseptic. Chewing on the tea tree leaves can provide many of the benefits that are experienced through the oil, and the leaves have been used in the past for the treatment of headaches. It can easily be grown indoors and in the right climate, it is an excellent outdoor plant as well.

Echinacea – Although there are many plants that are used for their healing properties in traditional Chinese medicine and elsewhere throughout the world, you will have a difficult time finding one that is more important than Echinacea. This herb can help to boost the immune system, allowing your own defenses to take care of bacterial and viral infections. Native Americans have also used this plant in times past for everything from snakebites to insect stings. It is easy to grow in soil that is fertile and well drained, but it does enjoy a lot of sunlight. Having fresh Echinacea is a much better choice than the store-bought options that are typically available.

Ginseng - This herb is grown for a wide variety of purposes, and it is likely that you will want to include it in your own garden as well. It can be used for a wide variety of healing purposes, and it also works as an aphrodisiac. Some of the specific reasons why you would use ginseng include for the healing of hypertension, symptoms related to menopause and erectile dysfunction.

Bupleurum - This plant can be used for many purposes, and it is a very strong cleansing agent that will clean the liver of many difficulties. It is also used in the treatment of ulcers, arthritis and may be able to help with emotional and mental problems. The plant has a relatively short growing season and you can sow the seeds in fertile soil, provided it is in full sun. If you're going to use it regularly, you can also grow it in pots indoors.

Chamomile - Most of us have enjoyed a cup of chamomile tea at some time in the past. It can certainly help to relax us when we are under stress and need to rest. Not only is it a delicious way to enjoy a cup of tea, it also provides a degree of aromatherapy that can help to reduce stress as well. Although most people don't realize it, chamomile is also used for the treatment of digestive problems and pain, including earaches and toothaches. It is easy to grow outdoors; the seeds can simply be broadcasted across a large area and the plants will grow quite well on their own.

Chinese Yam – This is a plant that can be easily grown in most areas, provided you have well-drained soil and plenty of sun. Once it is harvested, it can be consumed raw and may provide a number of healing benefits. It is a plant that has been used in traditional Chinese medicine for thousands of years. Some of the benefits that you may experience when eating the Chinese yam include those for the spleen and stomach, helping with poor digestion and even aiding weight loss. You may experience additional energy and it can even help with respiratory problems, such as a dry cough or asthma. This plant can also be applied externally for the treatment of abscesses, ulcers and boils.

Sea Buckthorn – This plant has been used in traditional Chinese medicine for thousands of years for the treatment of many different issues that you may be facing. It may be beneficial for digestive purposes, for reducing a problem with coughing and to aid in circulatory difficulties. At times, it has been used to reduce pain as well. The plant is also rather diverse, with the leaves and bark being used for gastrointestinal problems or topically for the treatment of arthritis. The berries, however, can be made into a juice and used for the healing of many different problems, including liver disease, cancer and ulcers.

Licorice Root - This plant has quite a few healing properties and it is something that you may want to consider growing in your garden. It tends to grow well in warmer climates when the soil is fertile, deep and drains well. It is also grown in full sun, so you don't want to shade the plant. It does take a while for it to grow, however, and after planting it, you will not be able to harvest it for approximately three years. The licorice root can be made into a healing tea and is used for many purposes, including menstrual cramps, heartburn, menopause symptoms and even for treating the flu.

Ginger - Not only is this plant used for the taste that it provides to the food you are eating, it is also excellent for the digestion and can treat a case of diarrhea. It has also been used for circulatory difficulties and for individuals who have problems with their heart. You can grow ginger very easily. Simply purchase some organic ginger, preferably in the spring, and bury it in some fertile soil. It can also easily be grown in a pot on the windowsill. It is one of the easiest plants to grow because it doesn't take much attention in order to grow heartily.

Ma Huang - This herb has been used in traditional Chinese medicine for thousands of years. It can be used for many different purposes, as is the case with many herbs that are used for medicinal reasons. Some of the more specific reasons why Ma Huang is used include for the treatment of hay fever, asthma, and it may help to treat the common cold as well. You can purchase the seeds and grow them yourself, but you will likely need to sprout them indoors or in a greenhouse. It takes several years of growth before you are able to harvest it but the healing properties of this herb make it well worth the wait.

Marsh Mallow - Although this plant is best known because it was used in the making of marshmallows, it has been used for thousands of years by many cultures because of its healing properties as well. Some of its uses include the treatment of sore throats, coughing, and indigestion. It may also have anti-inflammatory properties. This plant is relatively easy to grow, provided you live in the right climate. It tends to grow well in zones 3-9 and it is a perennial that loves rich soil and full sun.

Marigold - Although most people don't realize it, marigolds have been used successfully for many different medicinal purposes for years. It is typically considered to be somewhat of a common flower and is inexpensive to purchase in most areas where it grows readily. Applied externally, it can be used for the treatment of wounds, stings, sprains and even for varicose veins. It is also possible to make a tea from the petals that can be used for varicose veins and can improve circulation.

Aloe Vera - Every home should have at least one aloe vera plant available, and if possible, multiple plants both indoors and outdoors. It is an excellent choice for growth at home because it can help with the healing process when you experience any type of cut, and it is great to put on a burn. You can also make a juice out of the mixture and it may be able to help with a wide variety of internal problems, including constipation, colitis and digestive upset. This plant will grow heartily on its own if the climate is right. It will also grow quite easily on the windowsill in almost any area.

This is just a sampling of some of the many plants that are used around the world for their healing properties. As you can tell, there are options available for almost any problem that you may be experiencing. Growing and using these herbs and other plants may provide you with the greatest benefit, because you can control the quality of what you are using.

6. Where to Buy What You Can't Grow

Ideally, it would be best if you were able to grow all of your own medicinal plants and to have them available for your use straight from the garden. Unfortunately, that is not always possible, but many of the plants that you can't grow at home are still readily available if they are purchased through the proper outlet. Making the right choices in this regard can assist you in taking the high quality herbs and natural supplements that you need for the healing properties that they contain.

Before we begin to talk about choosing high quality supplements from a commercial standpoint, it is important to recognize that you must look beyond the advertising efforts of many of the larger companies. In some cases, they may make it seem as if you're getting the highest quality product but in reality, you are getting something that is very low quality in comparison with what 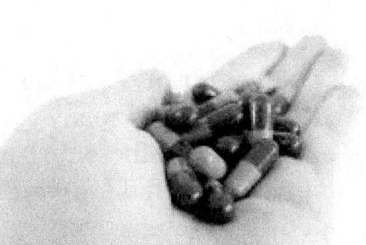 you would grow at home. The FDA does not regulate the vitamin and supplement industry in the same way that it regulates prescription drugs. It is necessary for you to be very cautious when choosing any natural treatment options, because you must be your own advocate.

You should also understand that I am not going to advocate one specific company or resource that you should be using. This is a very important decision to make, and you should look at your options and decide which one is best for your needs.

There is an old saying that you should not judge a book by its cover, and it is especially true to keep that in mind when you are dealing with supplements. On the outside, many supplements will look as if they are exactly what you need, and they may dazzle you with false advertising, using words such as all natural or organic. As we stated earlier, the FDA does not regulate what goes into these foods, so you are really on your own when it comes to choosing one that will be right for your needs. This would also include the statements as to what may be inside of the product. Unfortunately, you cannot determine if you are getting the true ingredients that you want by simply looking at the label.

It is important, however, for you to read the labels carefully and to try to determine what is inside of the product. At the very least, it should use an organic resource for the ingredients that are included. Look for any type of additional substances that may be included in the product, some of which may be hidden behind unusually descriptive words. If you have any questions as to what one of the ingredients is, you can research it online.

It is also important to check the expiration date on the product and to choose one that is relatively fresh. Of course, this is another area that is somewhat gray, but it may help to clear up some of the questions that you have about the product.

Don't underestimate the benefit of checking for reviews of the product online. It is likely that you will find many reviews of various products, some of which are positive and others that may be negative. I tend to throw out the best and the worst and look for the truth, that tends to fall somewhere in the middle. I am also very cautious about any flowery reviews that sound as if they come from somebody who is actually working for the company.

It can be difficult to find a high quality resource where you can buy your supplements but once you find one, make sure that you use them consistently. The benefits that are provided through the supplements that you take are something that will follow you for many years. Even though it may be best to grow your own medicinal food and herbs, when you have to buy them, make sure you are buying quality.

7. Living a Healthier Lifestyle

The bulk of this publication has been about growing and using medicinal plants as part of traditional Chinese medicine. If you do so, it may be possible for you to treat your health in an amazing way, and it is difficult to say where you may be able to go from here. In reality, the Chinese are not only famous for herbology and understanding how plants affect our health; they are also well versed in other factors that can make you healthy. The following information can assist you in living a healthier lifestyle and in doing so according to ancient principles.

Considering Your Diet First

The first thing that should be considered in any healthy lifestyle is your diet. Unfortunately, many of us tend to eat what has come to be known

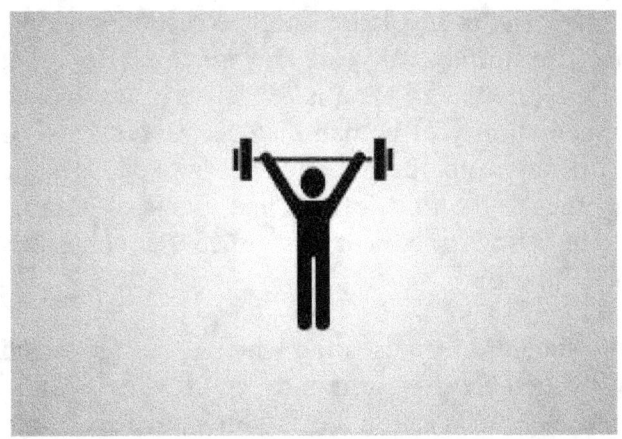

as the standard American diet, and it is one of the unhealthiest ways for us to eat. It is full of unnatural, unhealthy fats and is typically very high in sugar and other fast carbohydrates. If you want to affect your health in a positive way, you need to make changes in your diet first.

It can be difficult to choose a diet that is right for you. After all, at no point in history have there been so many options available for how we can eat. You have everything from low-fat to low carbohydrate and a wide variety of commercial weight loss programs that flood the supermarkets and late-night infomercials. Although many of these diets can help you to a certain extent in losing weight, that is not the entire battle. Yes, it is important to maintain a healthy weight but you need to be healthy on the inside as well as the outside.

First of all, it is important to recognize that almost every diet today is not following the basic principles of traditional Chinese medicine. Most of them tend to focus too much on meat, and even if you are not eating meat as part of your diet, it is likely that you are trying to limit the amount of fat that you are eating or perhaps limit your carbohydrates. In either case, you are missing out on one of the most beneficial ways of eating, one that is very similar to the way that someone in China thousands of years ago would have eaten.

It is not only the Chinese that understand the basic principles of how to eat healthily, many societies around the world eat a similar way, although the food may vary from one society to another. In any case, it is a diet that is based largely on starch, is fairly low or perhaps even does not include any meat and has a healthy portion of fruits and vegetables on the side. Why is it so important to eat this way?

When you do any research on dieting, you are likely to read that people have been hunter gatherers for millions of years and we come from that type of civilization. In reality, however, meat is a relative newcomer to the human diet, and for the majority of human history, we got most of our calories and our nutrition from the starches that we ate. In the Chinese culture, starch comes in the form of rice and this is something that is consumed in large quantities at almost every meal. How has this affected the health of the Chinese?

An individual that eats the standard Chinese diet, which is high in starch and includes fruits and vegetables, is going to be a very healthy individual. It is only because of the Western diets, which have crept into the Chinese culture, that the Chinese have become unhealthy as a group. In fact, many people from China that come to the United States are trim but when they begin to incorporate the standard American diet, they begin to gain weight and soon they are overweight and out of shape.

A diet does not need to be a complex factor in our life. In fact, if you just follow the basic principles of a diet that is based on starch, you will find that you are a much healthier individual. Cut out the sugars, wheat and boxed/canned food and opt for a diet that contains a lot of starch, such as rice, potatoes and corn. You can also eat a little bit of meat on the side if you prefer, but try to choose a healthier option, such as chicken, turkey or fish. Include some fruits and vegetables with your meals and snack on fruit if you have a sweet tooth.

What is the benefit of eating a diet that is based on starch? First of all, it is going to allow your body to seek a balance in a number of ways. You will find that you are losing weight quickly and are able to maintain a healthy weight for the rest of your life. Additionally, many of the foods that we eat on the standard American diet lead to inflammation and disease. When you base your diet on starch, fruits and vegetables, you will find that you are reducing many of the problems in your life, including hypertension, diabetes and other similar difficulties.

Don't Forget to Exercise

It is also very important that you get some exercise on a regular basis. The type of exercise that you get may vary according to your circumstances, but you can learn a lot about the way that the ancient Chinese exercised. In part, they got a lot of their exercise from the work that they did in the fields, but today we tend to work under fluorescent skies while sitting behind a computer. With a little bit of effort on your part, however, you can get a healthy amount of exercise that would amount to approximately 20-30 minutes per day.

There are many different ways that you can exercise, and it doesn't need to be something that is overly complex. Simply walking around the block a few times or perhaps jumping on a rebounder can help to build up your overall level of health and provide you with additional energy and the other benefits that exercise has to offer. When you incorporate exercise into your daily routine, you will prosper from it.

Stay Hydrated

It is also very important to make sure that you are staying hydrated on a regular basis. Chronic dehydration is a problem for millions of people around the world, but if you have access to clean drinking water, make sure that you are taking advantage of it.

One of the questions that many people have about drinking water is in regards to the type of water that they should be drinking. In fact, some people even avoid drinking water because they don't have a high quality water filter. It is much better for you to drink tap water and stay hydrated than to be dehydrated because you are avoiding drinking water.

How much water should you drink every day? Typically, the average person would need approximately 3 quarts of water daily. You can also drink more, if desired, but don't drink gallons of water at a time, thinking that it will help you to stay hydrated. Drink enough water throughout the day to keep your thirst at a minimum or to make it nonexistent. Drinking too much water can deplete your electrolytes, but drinking enough water will help you to maintain your health.

Pay Attention to Your Stress Levels

One other factor that you can consider for maintaining a healthy lifestyle is to lower your stress levels to the greatest extent possible. This is also something that is part of traditional Chinese medicine, and it is usually found in the form of yoga or meditation. You can take a page out of this book and improve your health as well.

It is not necessary for you to meditate for hours on end in order to benefit from it. In fact, just sitting quietly in a room for a few minutes a day is all that is typically necessary to reset your senses and to enjoy the benefits of what meditation has to offer. Additionally, you can do some stretching on a daily basis and some deep breathing exercises. It will help to keep your body in shape and will reduce your stress significantly.

These are just a few of the factors that can help you to be healthier and happier while at the same time, following the basics of traditional Chinese medicine. Remember that the road to health is one that takes some time to travel and it is really the small battles that will make a difference, if you win them consistently. Pay attention to all aspects of your life and you will be able to enjoy good health for a very long time.

8. Other Healing Options in Chinese Medicine

Although it certainly is true that eating properly can help to boost your health in numerous ways, there are also some other factors that you can consider for increasing your health through traditional Chinese medicine. In this chapter, we are going to take a look at a few of the additional factors that can help you to get more out of your health by incorporating the right things into your life.

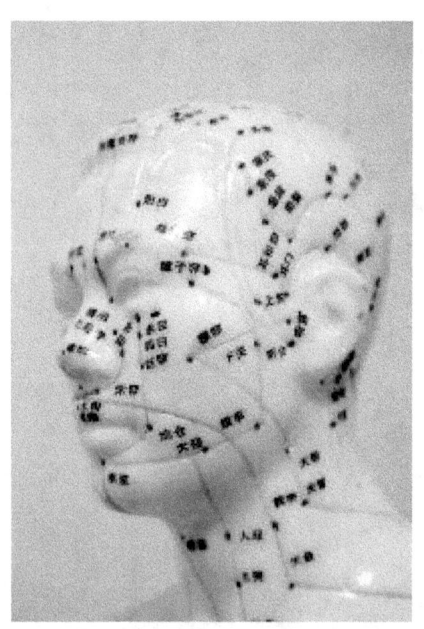

Acupuncture – This is a form of ancient Chinese medicine that has been practiced for thousands of years. According to the principles of acupuncture, small needles are inserted into specific areas of the body that will affect the flow of energy (Qi) in the body along the meridians. If, at any time, the energy within the body is not flowing properly, it will result in problems that are experienced either mentally or physically.

For example, the flow of energy along the meridians will help to keep the body in balance and will allow you to experience a higher level of energy, peace of mind and better physical health. When the energy is blocked, however, it may lead to problems such as pain, disease or mental problems. Rather than simply providing you with a prescription drug that would fight the symptoms, acupuncture looks to the source of the problem and tries to restore the free flow of energy again.

Acupuncture is a form of alternative therapy, and it is still practiced down to this day. In many cases, the practitioner that is providing acupuncture treatments for you is going to use the same basic principles of acupuncture that have been the hallmark of the treatment for thousands of years. People use acupuncture for a wide variety of purposes, from treating pain and disease to helping with weight loss or even to quitting smoking.

Massage – Another type of traditional Chinese therapy is to use massage as a form of healing. Massage is very similar to acupuncture, in that it helps to provide the free flow of energy throughout the body. The difference between massage and acupuncture is the way in which the energy is manipulated.

The masseuse will use his or her hands, arms, elbows, shoulders and other body parts to work with your body so that the energy is able to flow freely. This is not only true when it comes to the energy within your body directly; it is also thought that energy comes from the individual providing the massage that can help you to overcome a wide variety of problems as well.

There may also be certain types of massage that are specific to certain parts of the world. For example, Thai massage is very different from a traditional massage, and it provides very specific benefits. In some cases, a masseuse will travel to the area of the world where the type of massage that they are practicing originated in order to learn more about it. When they do so, they are keeping with the ancient practice and providing a more specific and beneficial experience to their customers.

9. Healing Herbs and Tea FAQ

In this publication, we have provided you with much information on how to grow your own medicinal herbs and how to use them more effectively. In this chapter, we are going to answer some more specific questions that many people have about the use of herbs and tea for healing. Some of these have been answered in other places of this publication but they are provided here for an easier reference.

Q: How quickly will herbs work for treating my physical problems?

A: If there is one thing that modern medicine has taught us, it is to expect something to happen immediately. Unfortunately, many of the benefits that are provided from modern medicine are only for the treatment of symptoms and not for a cure. Consider the fact that your disease did not happen overnight and it may have taken decades of poor health and a poor lifestyle to reach this point in your life. When you begin to use herbs and other food for healing, you may be able to experience some benefits quickly but ultimately, it is going to take perseverance on your part in order to see it through to its finality.

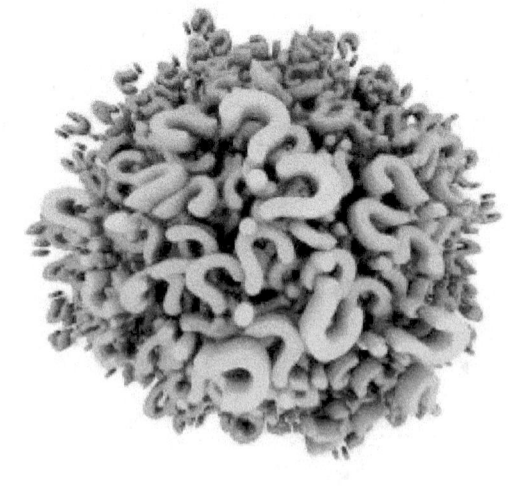

Q: Are there any problems associated with using herbs and other food for healing?

A: By and large, it is possible for you to use herbs and other types of food without any serious difficulties. Side effects are much lighter or perhaps nonexistent in comparison to what you may experience by using prescription medicine or other offerings through modern medical practices. There may be some issues that are associated with using herbs and food, however, that can include allergic reactions and interactions with medication that you may be taking. That is why it is important for you to discuss your use of herbs and other natural forms of treatment with your physician.

Q: What if I cannot grow my own herbs?

A: Almost all of us can grow at least some herbs, because it is possible to grow them on a windowsill in your home. It may be, however, that you are unable to grow the specific herbs that are necessary for your health problem. If that is the case, you can purchase high quality commercial supplements but only after you have confirmed that they are from a company you can trust.